CW00728279

Ketogenic

MEATS

- Beef
- Sausage
- Bacon
- Lamb
- Pork
- Veal
- Chicken/Turkey
- Eggs

VEGGIES

- Avocado
- Asparagus
- Argula
- Broccoli
- Cauliflower
- Brussel Sprouts
- Cabbage
- Celery

VEGGIES

- Cucumber
- Chards
- Bell Peppers
- Green Beans
- Collards
- Mushrooms
- Spinach
- Olives

FRUITS

- Blackberries
- Cranberries
- Blueberries
- Lemon
- Lime
- Raspberries
- Strawberries
- Plantains (paleo)

DAIRY

- Cheese (all kinds)
- Sour Cream
- Cream Cheese
- Heavy Cream
- Greek Yogurt
- Almond Milk
- Cashew Milk
- Coconut Cream

CONDIMENTS

- Balsamic Vinegar
- Beef/Chicken Broth
- Bonito Flakes
- Tartar Sauce (keto)
- Dijon Mustard
- Mayo
- Low Sugar Ketchup
- Pickles

OILS & FATS

- Avocado Oil
- Butter
- Coconut Butter
- Duck Fat
- Lard/Ghee
- Nut Oils
- Olive Oil
- Pork Rinds

HERBS & SPICES

- Garlic
- Salt & Pepper
- Oregano
- Paprika
- Cumin
- Chili Pepper
- Basil
- Ginger

BAKING

- Almond Flour
- Almond Meal
- Cashew Flour
- Oat Fiber
- Psyllium Husk
- Whey Protein
- Flax meal
- Hazelnut Flour

FISH/SEAFOOD

- Anchovy
- Haddock / Cod
- Halibut
- Crab/Lobster
- Mackerel
- Salmon
- Tuna
- Red Snapper

DRINKS

- Diet Soda (moderation)
- Coffee
- Tea
- Gatorade Zero
- Protein Shake
- Club Soda
- Broth
- Coconut Water

MISC.

- Canned Tuna
- Pesto
- Soy Sauce
- Aioli
- Béarnaise
- Vinaigrette
- Hot Sauce
- Guacamole

NOTES:

Weekly Meal Planner

Week of: _____

	Breakfast	Lunch	Dinner	Snack	Notes
Monday	TOTAL Carbs Fat Protein Cals	TOTAL Carbs Fat Protein Cals	TOTAL Carbs Fat Protein Cals	TOTAL Carbs Fat Protein Cals	
Tuesday	TOTAL Carbs Fat Protein Cals	TOTAL Carbs Fat Protein Cals	TOTAL Carbs Fat Protein Cals	TOTAL Carbs Fat Protein Cals	
Wednesday	TOTAL Carbs Fa Protein Cals	TOTAL Carbs Fat Protein Cals	TOTAL Carbs Fat Protein Cals	TOTAL Carbs Fat Protein Cals	
Thursday	TOTAL Carbs Fa Protein Cals	TOTAL Carbs Fat Protein Cals	TOTAL Carbs Fat Protein Cals	TOTAL Carbs Fat Protein Cals	
Friday	TOTAL Carbs Fa Protein Cals	TOTAL Carbs Fat Protein Cals	TOTAL Carbs Fat Protein Cals	TOTAL Carbs Fat Protein Cals	
Saturday	TOTAL Carbs Fa Protein Cals	TOTAL Carbs Fat Protein Cals	TOTAL Carbs Fat Protein Cals	TOTAL Carbs Fat Protein Cals	
Sunday	TOTAL Carbs Fa Protein Cals	TOTAL Carbs Fat Protein Cals	TOTAL Carbs Fat Protein Cals	TOTAL Carbs Fat Protein Cals	

Keto Grocery Inventory

DATE: _____

QTY	PRODUCE

QTY	MEAT & FISH

QTY	FROZEN FOODS

QTY	DAIRY

QTY	PANTRY

QTY	OTHER/MISC.

Low Carb Grocery Ideas

FRESH PRODUCE

Asparagus	Cauliflower	Onions
Avocado	Celery	Radishes
Bell Peppers	Cucumber	Salad Mix
Berries	Eggplant	Squash
Broccoli	Fennel	Tomatoes
Brussel Sprouts	Garlic	Bok Choi
Cabbage	Green Beans	Chives
Carrots	Mushrooms	Spinach

MEAT AND SEAFOOD

Bacon	Lamb	Fish
Beef	Pork	Crab
Bison	Rotisserie Chicken	Lobster
Chicken	Sausage	Scallops
Deli meat	Turkey	Shrimp
Ground Beef / Ground Turkey	Oyster	Mussels

DAIRY PRODUCTS

Butter	Eggs	Sour Cream
Cheese	Greek Yogurt, full fat	Ghee
Cream Cheese	Heavy Whipping Cream	Mayo

PANTRY ITEMS

Avocado oil	Tea/Coffee	Moon Cheese
Beef Jerky	Pork Rinds	Low Carb Protein Bars
Bone Broth	Mayonnaise	All Natural Peanut Butter
Tuna, Salmon (canned)	Low Carb Salad Dressing	Stevia
Coconut Butter	Olive oil, extra virgin	Almonds
Coconut Oil	Olives	Spices
Almond Milk	Sweeteners	Almond Flour

FROZEN / OTHER

Low Carb Shopping List

FRESH PRODUCE

MEAT AND SEAFOOD

DAIRY PRODUCTS

PANTRY ITEMS

FROZEN / OTHER

Weekly Meal Planner

Week of: _____

	Breakfast	Lunch	Dinner	Snack	Notes
Monday	Carbs Fat Protein TOTAL Cals	Carbs Fat Protein TOTAL Cals	Carbs Fat Protein TOTAL Cals	Carbs Fat Protein TOTAL Cals	
Tuesday	Carbs Fat Protein TOTAL Cals	Carbs Fat Protein TOTAL Cals	Carbs Fat Protein TOTAL Cals	Carbs Fat Protein TOTAL Cals	
Wednesday	Carbs Fat Protein TOTAL Cals	Carbs Fat Protein TOTAL Cals	Carbs Fat Protein TOTAL Cals	Carbs Fat Protein TOTAL Cals	
Thursday	Carbs Fat Protein TOTAL Cals	Carbs Fat Protein TOTAL Cals	Carbs Fat Protein TOTAL Cals	Carbs Fat Protein TOTAL Cals	
Friday	Carbs Fat Protein TOTAL Cals	Carbs Fat Protein TOTAL Cals	Carbs Fat Protein TOTAL Cals	Carbs Fat Protein TOTAL Cals	
Saturday	Carbs Fat Protein TOTAL Cals	Carbs Fat Protein TOTAL Cals	Carbs Fat Protein TOTAL Cals	Carbs Fat Protein TOTAL Cals	
Sunday	Carbs Fat Protein TOTAL Cals	Carbs Fat Protein TOTAL Cals	Carbs Fat Protein TOTAL Cals	Carbs Fat Protein TOTAL Cals	

Keto Grocery Inventory

DATE: _____

QTY	PRODUCE

QTY	MEAT & FISH

QTY	FROZEN FOODS

QTY	DAIRY

QTY	PANTRY

QTY	OTHER/MISC.

Low Carb Grocery Ideas

FRESH PRODUCE

☐ Asparagus	☐ Cauliflower	☐ Onions
☐ Avocado	☐ Celery	☐ Radishes
☐ Bell Peppers	☐ Cucumber	☐ Salad Mix
☐ Berries	☐ Eggplant	☐ Squash
☐ Broccoli	☐ Fennel	☐ Tomatoes
☐ Brussel Sprouts	☐ Garlic	☐ Bok Choi
☐ Cabbage	☐ Green Beans	☐ Chives
☐ Carrots	☐ Mushrooms	☐ Spinach

MEAT AND SEAFOOD

☐ Bacon	☐ Lamb	☐ Fish
☐ Beef	☐ Pork	☐ Crab
☐ Bison	☐ Rotisserie Chicken	☐ Lobster
☐ Chicken	☐ Sausage	☐ Scallops
☐ Deli meat	☐ Turkey	☐ Shrimp
☐ Ground Beef / Ground Turkey	☐ Oyster	☐ Mussels

DAIRY PRODUCTS

☐ Butter	☐ Eggs	☐ Sour Cream
☐ Cheese	☐ Greek Yogurt, full fat	☐ Ghee
☐ Cream Cheese	☐ Heavy Whipping Cream	☐ Mayo

PANTRY ITEMS

☐ Avocado oil	☐ Tea/Coffee	☐ Moon Cheese
☐ Beef Jerky	☐ Pork Rinds	☐ Low Carb Protein Bars
☐ Bone Broth	☐ Mayonnaise	☐ All Natural Peanut Butter
☐ Tuna, Salmon (canned)	☐ Low Carb Salad Dressing	☐ Stevia
☐ Coconut Butter	☐ Olive oil, extra virgin	☐ Almonds
☐ Coconut Oil	☐ Olives	☐ Spices
☐ Almond Milk	☐ Sweeteners	☐ Almond Flour

FROZEN / OTHER

☐	☐	☐
☐	☐	☐
☐	☐	☐
☐	☐	☐

Low Carb Shopping List

FRESH PRODUCE

MEAT AND SEAFOOD

DAIRY PRODUCTS

PANTRY ITEMS

FROZEN / OTHER

Weekly Meal Planner

Week of: _____

	Breakfast	Lunch	Dinner	Snack	Notes
Monday	Carbs Fat Protein TOTAL Cals	Carbs Fat Protein TOTAL Cals	Carbs Fat Protein TOTAL Cals	Carbs Fat Protein TOTAL Cals	
Tuesday	Carbs Fat Protein TOTAL Cals	Carbs Fat Protein TOTAL Cals	Carbs Fat Protein TOTAL Cals	Carbs Fat Protein TOTAL Cals	
Wednesday	Carbs Fat Protein TOTAL Cals	Carbs Fat Protein TOTAL Cals	Carbs Fat Protein TOTAL Cals	Carbs Fat Protein TOTAL Cals	
Thursday	Carbs Fat Protein TOTAL Cals	Carbs Fat Protein TOTAL Cals	Carbs Fat Protein TOTAL Cals	Carbs Fat Protein TOTAL Cals	
Friday	Carbs Fat Protein TOTAL Cals	Carbs Fat Protein TOTAL Cals	Carbs Fat Protein TOTAL Cals	Carbs Fat Protein TOTAL Cals	
Saturday	Carbs Fat Protein TOTAL Cals	Carbs Fat Protein TOTAL Cals	Carbs Fat Protein TOTAL Cals	Carbs Fat Protein TOTAL Cals	
Sunday	Carbs Fat Protein TOTAL Cals	Carbs Fat Protein TOTAL Cals	Carbs Fat Protein TOTAL Cals	Carbs Fat Protein TOTAL Cals	

Keto Grocery Inventory

DATE: _____

QTY	PRODUCE

QTY	MEAT & FISH

QTY	FROZEN FOODS

QTY	DAIRY

QTY	PANTRY

QTY	OTHER/MISC.

Low Carb Grocery Ideas

FRESH PRODUCE

☐ Asparagus	☐ Cauliflower	☐ Onions
☐ Avocado	☐ Celery	☐ Radishes
☐ Bell Peppers	☐ Cucumber	☐ Salad Mix
☐ Berries	☐ Eggplant	☐ Squash
☐ Broccoli	☐ Fennel	☐ Tomatoes
☐ Brussel Sprouts	☐ Garlic	☐ Bok Choi
☐ Cabbage	☐ Green Beans	☐ Chives
☐ Carrots	☐ Mushrooms	☐ Spinach

MEAT AND SEAFOOD

☐ Bacon	☐ Lamb	☐ Fish
☐ Beef	☐ Pork	☐ Crab
☐ Bison	☐ Rotisserie Chicken	☐ Lobster
☐ Chicken	☐ Sausage	☐ Scallops
☐ Deli meat	☐ Turkey	☐ Shrimp
☐ Ground Beef / Ground Turkey	☐ Oyster	☐ Mussels

DAIRY PRODUCTS

☐ Butter	☐ Eggs	☐ Sour Cream
☐ Cheese	☐ Greek Yogurt, full fat	☐ Ghee
☐ Cream Cheese	☐ Heavy Whipping Cream	☐ Mayo

PANTRY ITEMS

☐ Avocado oil	☐ Tea/Coffee	☐ Moon Cheese
☐ Beef Jerky	☐ Pork Rinds	☐ Low Carb Protein Bars
☐ Bone Broth	☐ Mayonnaise	☐ All Natural Peanut Butter
☐ Tuna, Salmon (canned)	☐ Low Carb Salad Dressing	☐ Stevia
☐ Coconut Butter	☐ Olive oil, extra virgin	☐ Almonds
☐ Coconut Oil	☐ Olives	☐ Spices
☐ Almond Milk	☐ Sweeteners	☐ Almond Flour

FROZEN / OTHER

☐	☐	☐
☐	☐	☐
☐	☐	☐
☐	☐	☐

Low Carb Shopping List

FRESH PRODUCE

MEAT AND SEAFOOD

DAIRY PRODUCTS

PANTRY ITEMS

FROZEN / OTHER

Weekly Meal Planner

Week of: _____

	Breakfast	Lunch	Dinner	Snack	Notes
Monday	TOTAL Carbs Fat Protein Cals	TOTAL Carbs Fat Protein Cals	TOTAL Carbs Fa Protein Cals	TOTAL Carbs Fat Protein Cals	
Tuesday	TOTAL Carbs Fat Protein Cals	TOTAL Carbs Fat Protein Cals	TOTAL Carbs Fat Protein Cals	TOTAL Carbs Fat Protein Cals	
Wednesday	TOTAL Carbs Fa Protein Cals	TOTAL Carbs Fat Protein Cals	TOTAL Carbs Fat Protein Cals	TOTAL Carbs Fat Protein Cals	
Thursday	TOTAL Carbs Fa Protein Cals	TOTAL Carbs Fat Protein Cals	TOTAL Carbs Fat Protein Cals	TOTAL Carbs Fat Protein Cals	
Friday	TOTAL Carbs Fa Protein Cals	TOTAL Carbs Fat Protein Cals	TOTAL Carbs Fat Protein Cals	TOTAL Carbs Fat Protein Cals	
Saturday	TOTAL Carbs Fa Protein Cals	TOTAL Carbs Fat Protein Cals	TOTAL Carbs Fat Protein Cals	TOTAL Carbs Fat Protein Cals	
Sunday	TOTAL Carbs Fa Protein Cals	TOTAL Carbs Fat Protein Cals	TOTAL Carbs Fat Protein Cals	TOTAL Carbs Fat Protein Cals	

Keto Grocery Inventory

DATE: _____

QTY	PRODUCE

QTY	MEAT & FISH

QTY	FROZEN FOODS

QTY	DAIRY

QTY	PANTRY

QTY	OTHER/MISC.

Low Carb Grocery Ideas

FRESH PRODUCE

☐ Asparagus	☐ Cauliflower	☐ Onions
☐ Avocado	☐ Celery	☐ Radishes
☐ Bell Peppers	☐ Cucumber	☐ Salad Mix
☐ Berries	☐ Eggplant	☐ Squash
☐ Broccoli	☐ Fennel	☐ Tomatoes
☐ Brussel Sprouts	☐ Garlic	☐ Bok Choi
☐ Cabbage	☐ Green Beans	☐ Chives
☐ Carrots	☐ Mushrooms	☐ Spinach

MEAT AND SEAFOOD

☐ Bacon	☐ Lamb	☐ Fish
☐ Beef	☐ Pork	☐ Crab
☐ Bison	☐ Rotisserie Chicken	☐ Lobster
☐ Chicken	☐ Sausage	☐ Scallops
☐ Deli meat	☐ Turkey	☐ Shrimp
☐ Ground Beef / Ground Turkey	☐ Oyster	☐ Mussels

DAIRY PRODUCTS

☐ Butter	☐ Eggs	☐ Sour Cream
☐ Cheese	☐ Greek Yogurt, full fat	☐ Ghee
☐ Cream Cheese	☐ Heavy Whipping Cream	☐ Mayo

PANTRY ITEMS

☐ Avocado oil	☐ Tea/Coffee	☐ Moon Cheese
☐ Beef Jerky	☐ Pork Rinds	☐ Low Carb Protein Bars
☐ Bone Broth	☐ Mayonnaise	☐ All Natural Peanut Butter
☐ Tuna, Salmon (canned)	☐ Low Carb Salad Dressing	☐ Stevia
☐ Coconut Butter	☐ Olive oil, extra virgin	☐ Almonds
☐ Coconut Oil	☐ Olives	☐ Spices
☐ Almond Milk	☐ Sweeteners	☐ Almond Flour

FROZEN / OTHER

☐	☐	☐
☐	☐	☐
☐	☐	☐
☐	☐	☐

Low Carb Shopping List

FRESH PRODUCE

MEAT AND SEAFOOD

DAIRY PRODUCTS

PANTRY ITEMS

FROZEN / OTHER

Weekly Meal Planner

Week of: _____

	Breakfast	Lunch	Dinner	Snack	Notes
Monday	Carbs Fat Protein TOTAL Cals	Carbs Fat Protein TOTAL Cals	Carbs Fat Protein TOTAL Cals	Carbs Fat Protein TOTAL Cals	
Tuesday	Carbs Fat Protein TOTAL Cals	Carbs Fat Protein TOTAL Cals	Carbs Fat Protein TOTAL Cals	Carbs Fat Protein TOTAL Cals	
Wednesday	Carbs Fat Protein TOTAL Cals	Carbs Fat Protein TOTAL Cals	Carbs Fat Protein TOTAL Cals	Carbs Fat Protein TOTAL Cals	
Thursday	Carbs Fat Protein TOTAL Cals	Carbs Fat Protein TOTAL Cals	Carbs Fat Protein TOTAL Cals	Carbs Fat Protein TOTAL Cals	
Friday	Carbs Fat Protein TOTAL Cals	Carbs Fat Protein TOTAL Cals	Carbs Fat Protein TOTAL Cals	Carbs Fat Protein TOTAL Cals	
Saturday	Carbs Fat Protein TOTAL Cals	Carbs Fat Protein TOTAL Cals	Carbs Fat Protein TOTAL Cals	Carbs Fat Protein TOTAL Cals	
Sunday	Carbs Fat Protein TOTAL Cals	Carbs Fat Protein TOTAL Cals	Carbs Fat Protein TOTAL Cals	Carbs Fat Protein TOTAL Cals	

Keto Grocery Inventory

DATE: _____

QTY	PRODUCE

QTY	MEAT & FISH

QTY	FROZEN FOODS

QTY	DAIRY

QTY	PANTRY

QTY	OTHER/MISC.

Low Carb Grocery Ideas

FRESH PRODUCE

☐ Asparagus	☐ Cauliflower	☐ Onions
☐ Avocado	☐ Celery	☐ Radishes
☐ Bell Peppers	☐ Cucumber	☐ Salad Mix
☐ Berries	☐ Eggplant	☐ Squash
☐ Broccoli	☐ Fennel	☐ Tomatoes
☐ Brussel Sprouts	☐ Garlic	☐ Bok Choi
☐ Cabbage	☐ Green Beans	☐ Chives
☐ Carrots	☐ Mushrooms	☐ Spinach

MEAT AND SEAFOOD

☐ Bacon	☐ Lamb	☐ Fish
☐ Beef	☐ Pork	☐ Crab
☐ Bison	☐ Rotisserie Chicken	☐ Lobster
☐ Chicken	☐ Sausage	☐ Scallops
☐ Deli meat	☐ Turkey	☐ Shrimp
☐ Ground Beef / Ground Turkey	☐ Oyster	☐ Mussels

DAIRY PRODUCTS

☐ Butter	☐ Eggs	☐ Sour Cream
☐ Cheese	☐ Greek Yogurt, full fat	☐ Ghee
☐ Cream Cheese	☐ Heavy Whipping Cream	☐ Mayo

PANTRY ITEMS

☐ Avocado oil	☐ Tea/Coffee	☐ Moon Cheese
☐ Beef Jerky	☐ Pork Rinds	☐ Low Carb Protein Bars
☐ Bone Broth	☐ Mayonnaise	☐ All Natural Peanut Butter
☐ Tuna, Salmon (canned)	☐ Low Carb Salad Dressing	☐ Stevia
☐ Coconut Butter	☐ Olive oil, extra virgin	☐ Almonds
☐ Coconut Oil	☐ Olives	☐ Spices
☐ Almond Milk	☐ Sweeteners	☐ Almond Flour

FROZEN / OTHER

☐	☐	☐
☐	☐	☐
☐	☐	☐
☐	☐	☐

Low Carb Shopping List

FRESH PRODUCE

MEAT AND SEAFOOD

DAIRY PRODUCTS

PANTRY ITEMS

FROZEN / OTHER

Weekly Meal Planner

Week of: _____

	Breakfast	Lunch	Dinner	Snack	Notes
Monday	Carbs Fat Protein TOTAL Cals	Carbs Fat Protein TOTAL Cals	Carbs Fat Protein TOTAL Cals	Carbs Fat Protein TOTAL Cals	_____ _____ _____
Tuesday	Carbs Fat Protein TOTAL Cals	Carbs Fat Protein TOTAL Cals	Carbs Fat Protein TOTAL Cals	Carbs Fat Protein TOTAL Cals	_____ _____ _____ _____
Wednesday	Carbs Fat Protein TOTAL Cals	Carbs Fat Protein TOTAL Cals	Carbs Fat Protein TOTAL Cals	Carbs Fat Protein TOTAL Cals	_____ _____ _____
Thursday	Carbs Fat Protein TOTAL Cals	Carbs Fat Protein TOTAL Cals	Carbs Fat Protein TOTAL Cals	Carbs Fat Protein TOTAL Cals	_____ _____ _____ _____
Friday	Carbs Fat Protein TOTAL Cals	Carbs Fat Protein TOTAL Cals	Carbs Fat Protein TOTAL Cals	Carbs Fat Protein TOTAL Cals	_____ _____ _____
Saturday	Carbs Fat Protein TOTAL Cals	Carbs Fat Protein TOTAL Cals	Carbs Fat Protein TOTAL Cals	Carbs Fat Protein TOTAL Cals	_____ _____ _____ _____
Sunday	Carbs Fat Protein TOTAL Cals	Carbs Fat Protein TOTAL Cals	Carbs Fat Protein TOTAL Cals	Carbs Fat Protein TOTAL Cals	_____ _____ _____

Keto Grocery Inventory

DATE:

QTY	PRODUCE

QTY	MEAT & FISH

QTY	FROZEN FOODS

QTY	DAIRY

QTY	PANTRY

QTY	OTHER/MISC.

Low Carb Grocery Ideas

FRESH PRODUCE

☐ Asparagus	☐ Cauliflower	☐ Onions
☐ Avocado	☐ Celery	☐ Radishes
☐ Bell Peppers	☐ Cucumber	☐ Salad Mix
☐ Berries	☐ Eggplant	☐ Squash
☐ Broccoli	☐ Fennel	☐ Tomatoes
☐ Brussel Sprouts	☐ Garlic	☐ Bok Choi
☐ Cabbage	☐ Green Beans	☐ Chives
☐ Carrots	☐ Mushrooms	☐ Spinach

MEAT AND SEAFOOD

☐ Bacon	☐ Lamb	☐ Fish
☐ Beef	☐ Pork	☐ Crab
☐ Bison	☐ Rotisserie Chicken	☐ Lobster
☐ Chicken	☐ Sausage	☐ Scallops
☐ Deli meat	☐ Turkey	☐ Shrimp
☐ Ground Beef / Ground Turkey	☐ Oyster	☐ Mussels

DAIRY PRODUCTS

☐ Butter	☐ Eggs	☐ Sour Cream
☐ Cheese	☐ Greek Yogurt, full fat	☐ Ghee
☐ Cream Cheese	☐ Heavy Whipping Cream	☐ Mayo

PANTRY ITEMS

☐ Avocado oil	☐ Tea/Coffee	☐ Moon Cheese
☐ Beef Jerky	☐ Pork Rinds	☐ Low Carb Protein Bars
☐ Bone Broth	☐ Mayonnaise	☐ All Natural Peanut Butter
☐ Tuna, Salmon (canned)	☐ Low Carb Salad Dressing	☐ Stevia
☐ Coconut Butter	☐ Olive oil, extra virgin	☐ Almonds
☐ Coconut Oil	☐ Olives	☐ Spices
☐ Almond Milk	☐ Sweeteners	☐ Almond Flour

FROZEN / OTHER

☐	☐	☐
☐	☐	☐
☐	☐	☐
☐	☐	☐

Low Carb Shopping List

FRESH PRODUCE

MEAT AND SEAFOOD

DAIRY PRODUCTS

PANTRY ITEMS

FROZEN / OTHER

Weekly Meal Planner

Week of: _____

	Breakfast	Lunch	Dinner	Snack	Notes
Monday	TOTAL Carbs Fat Protein Cals	TOTAL Carbs Fat Protein Cals	TOTAL Carbs Fat Protein Cals	TOTAL Carbs Fat Protein Cals	
Tuesday	TOTAL Carbs Fat Protein Cals	TOTAL Carbs Fat Protein Cals	TOTAL Carbs Fat Protein Cals	TOTAL Carbs Fat Protein Cals	
Wednesday	TOTAL Carbs Fat Protein Cals	TOTAL Carbs Fat Protein Cals	TOTAL Carbs Fat Protein Cals	TOTAL Carbs Fat Protein Cals	
Thursday	TOTAL Carbs Fat Protein Cals	TOTAL Carbs Fat Protein Cals	TOTAL Carbs Fat Protein Cals	TOTAL Carbs Fat Protein Cals	
Friday	TOTAL Carbs Fat Protein Cals	TOTAL Carbs Fat Protein Cals	TOTAL Carbs Fat Protein Cals	TOTAL Carbs Fat Protein Cals	
Saturday	TOTAL Carbs Fat Protein Cals	TOTAL Carbs Fat Protein Cals	TOTAL Carbs Fat Protein Cals	TOTAL Carbs Fat Protein Cals	
Sunday	TOTAL Carbs Fat Protein Cals	TOTAL Carbs Fat Protein Cals	TOTAL Carbs Fat Protein Cals	TOTAL Carbs Fat Protein Cals	

Keto Grocery Inventory

DATE:

QTY	PRODUCE

QTY	MEAT & FISH

QTY	FROZEN FOODS

QTY	DAIRY

QTY	PANTRY

QTY	OTHER/MISC.

Low Carb Grocery Ideas

FRESH PRODUCE

☐	Asparagus	☐	Cauliflower	☐	Onions
☐	Avocado	☐	Celery	☐	Radishes
☐	Bell Peppers	☐	Cucumber	☐	Salad Mix
☐	Berries	☐	Eggplant	☐	Squash
☐	Broccoli	☐	Fennel	☐	Tomatoes
☐	Brussel Sprouts	☐	Garlic	☐	Bok Choi
☐	Cabbage	☐	Green Beans	☐	Chives
☐	Carrots	☐	Mushrooms	☐	Spinach

MEAT AND SEAFOOD

☐	Bacon	☐	Lamb	☐	Fish
☐	Beef	☐	Pork	☐	Crab
☐	Bison	☐	Rotisserie Chicken	☐	Lobster
☐	Chicken	☐	Sausage	☐	Scallops
☐	Deli meat	☐	Turkey	☐	Shrimp
☐	Ground Beef / Ground Turkey	☐	Oyster	☐	Mussels

DAIRY PRODUCTS

☐	Butter	☐	Eggs	☐	Sour Cream
☐	Cheese	☐	Greek Yogurt, full fat	☐	Ghee
☐	Cream Cheese	☐	Heavy Whipping Cream	☐	Mayo

PANTRY ITEMS

☐	Avocado oil	☐	Tea/Coffee	☐	Moon Cheese
☐	Beef Jerky	☐	Pork Rinds	☐	Low Carb Protein Bars
☐	Bone Broth	☐	Mayonnaise	☐	All Natural Peanut Butter
☐	Tuna, Salmon (canned)	☐	Low Carb Salad Dressing	☐	Stevia
☐	Coconut Butter	☐	Olive oil, extra virgin	☐	Almonds
☐	Coconut Oil	☐	Olives	☐	Spices
☐	Almond Milk	☐	Sweeteners	☐	Almond Flour

FROZEN / OTHER

☐		☐		☐	
☐		☐		☐	
☐		☐		☐	
☐		☐		☐	

Low Carb Shopping List

FRESH PRODUCE

MEAT AND SEAFOOD

DAIRY PRODUCTS

PANTRY ITEMS

FROZEN / OTHER

Weekly Meal Planner

Week of: _____

	Breakfast	Lunch	Dinner	Snack	Notes
Monday	TOTAL Carbs Fat Protein Cals	TOTAL Carbs Fat Protein Cals	TOTAL Carbs Fat Protein Cals	TOTAL Carbs Fat Protein Cals	_____ _____ _____ _____
Tuesday	TOTAL Carbs Fat Protein Cals	TOTAL Carbs Fat Protein Cals	TOTAL Carbs Fat Protein Cals	TOTAL Carbs Fat Protein Cals	_____ _____ _____ _____ _____
Wednesday	TOTAL Carbs Fat Protein Cals	TOTAL Carbs Fat Protein Cals	TOTAL Carbs Fat Protein Cals	TOTAL Carbs Fat Protein Cals	_____ _____ _____ _____
Thursday	TOTAL Carbs Fat Protein Cals	TOTAL Carbs Fat Protein Cals	TOTAL Carbs Fat Protein Cals	TOTAL Carbs Fat Protein Cals	_____ _____ _____ _____
Friday	TOTAL Carbs Fat Protein Cals	TOTAL Carbs Fat Protein Cals	TOTAL Carbs Fat Protein Cals	TOTAL Carbs Fat Protein Cals	_____ _____ _____ _____
Saturday	TOTAL Carbs Fat Protein Cals	TOTAL Carbs Fat Protein Cals	TOTAL Carbs Fat Protein Cals	TOTAL Carbs Fat Protein Cals	_____ _____ _____ _____
Sunday	TOTAL Carbs Fat Protein Cals	TOTAL Carbs Fat Protein Cals	TOTAL Carbs Fat Protein Cals	TOTAL Carbs Fat Protein Cals	_____ _____ _____ _____

Keto Grocery Inventory

DATE: _____

QTY	PRODUCE

QTY	MEAT & FISH

QTY	FROZEN FOODS

QTY	DAIRY

QTY	PANTRY

QTY	OTHER/MISC.

Low Carb Grocery Ideas

FRESH PRODUCE

Asparagus	Cauliflower	Onions
Avocado	Celery	Radishes
Bell Peppers	Cucumber	Salad Mix
Berries	Eggplant	Squash
Broccoli	Fennel	Tomatoes
Brussel Sprouts	Garlic	Bok Choi
Cabbage	Green Beans	Chives
Carrots	Mushrooms	Spinach

MEAT AND SEAFOOD

Bacon	Lamb	Fish
Beef	Pork	Crab
Bison	Rotisserie Chicken	Lobster
Chicken	Sausage	Scallops
Deli meat	Turkey	Shrimp
Ground Beef / Ground Turkey	Oyster	Mussels

DAIRY PRODUCTS

Butter	Eggs	Sour Cream
Cheese	Greek Yogurt, full fat	Ghee
Cream Cheese	Heavy Whipping Cream	Mayo

PANTRY ITEMS

Avocado oil	Tea/Coffee	Moon Cheese
Beef Jerky	Pork Rinds	Low Carb Protein Bars
Bone Broth	Mayonnaise	All Natural Peanut Butter
Tuna, Salmon (canned)	Low Carb Salad Dressing	Stevia
Coconut Butter	Olive oil, extra virgin	Almonds
Coconut Oil	Olives	Spices
Almond Milk	Sweeteners	Almond Flour

FROZEN / OTHER

Low Carb Shopping List

FRESH PRODUCE

MEAT AND SEAFOOD

DAIRY PRODUCTS

PANTRY ITEMS

FROZEN / OTHER

Weekly Meal Planner

Week of: _____

	Breakfast	Lunch	Dinner	Snack	Notes
Monday					
	Carbs Fat Protein TOTAL Cals	Carbs Fat Protein TOTAL Cals	Carbs Fat Protein TOTAL Cals	Carbs Fat Protein TOTAL Cals	
Tuesday					
	Carbs Fat Protein TOTAL Cals	Carbs Fat Protein TOTAL Cals	Carbs Fat Protein TOTAL Cals	Carbs Fat Protein TOTAL Cals	
Wednesday					
	Carbs Fa Protein TOTAL Cals	Carbs Fat Protein TOTAL Cals	Carbs Fat Protein TOTAL Cals	Carbs Fat Protein TOTAL Cals	
Thursday					
	Carbs Fa Protein TOTAL Cals	Carbs Fat Protein TOTAL Cals	Carbs Fat Protein TOTAL Cals	Carbs Fat Protein TOTAL Cals	
Friday					
	Carbs Fa Protein TOTAL Cals	Carbs Fat Protein TOTAL Cals	Carbs Fat Protein TOTAL Cals	Carbs Fat Protein TOTAL Cals	
Saturday					
	Carbs Fa Protein TOTAL Cals	Carbs Fat Protein TOTAL Cals	Carbs Fat Protein TOTAL Cals	Carbs Fat Protein TOTAL Cals	
Sunday					
	Carbs Fa Protein TOTAL Cals	Carbs Fat Protein TOTAL Cals	Carbs Fat Protein TOTAL Cals	Carbs Fat Protein TOTAL Cals	

Keto Grocery Inventory

QTY	PRODUCE

QTY	MEAT & FISH

QTY	FROZEN FOODS

QTY	DAIRY

QTY	PANTRY

QTY	OTHER/MISC.

Low Carb Grocery Ideas

FRESH PRODUCE

☐ Asparagus	☐ Cauliflower	☐ Onions
☐ Avocado	☐ Celery	☐ Radishes
☐ Bell Peppers	☐ Cucumber	☐ Salad Mix
☐ Berries	☐ Eggplant	☐ Squash
☐ Broccoli	☐ Fennel	☐ Tomatoes
☐ Brussel Sprouts	☐ Garlic	☐ Bok Choi
☐ Cabbage	☐ Green Beans	☐ Chives
☐ Carrots	☐ Mushrooms	☐ Spinach

MEAT AND SEAFOOD

☐ Bacon	☐ Lamb	☐ Fish
☐ Beef	☐ Pork	☐ Crab
☐ Bison	☐ Rotisserie Chicken	☐ Lobster
☐ Chicken	☐ Sausage	☐ Scallops
☐ Deli meat	☐ Turkey	☐ Shrimp
☐ Ground Beef / Ground Turkey	☐ Oyster	☐ Mussels

DAIRY PRODUCTS

☐ Butter	☐ Eggs	☐ Sour Cream
☐ Cheese	☐ Greek Yogurt, full fat	☐ Ghee
☐ Cream Cheese	☐ Heavy Whipping Cream	☐ Mayo

PANTRY ITEMS

☐ Avocado oil	☐ Tea/Coffee	☐ Moon Cheese
☐ Beef Jerky	☐ Pork Rinds	☐ Low Carb Protein Bars
☐ Bone Broth	☐ Mayonnaise	☐ All Natural Peanut Butter
☐ Tuna, Salmon (canned)	☐ Low Carb Salad Dressing	☐ Stevia
☐ Coconut Butter	☐ Olive oil, extra virgin	☐ Almonds
☐ Coconut Oil	☐ Olives	☐ Spices
☐ Almond Milk	☐ Sweeteners	☐ Almond Flour

FROZEN / OTHER

☐	☐	☐
☐	☐	☐
☐	☐	☐
☐	☐	☐

Low Carb Shopping List

FRESH PRODUCE

MEAT AND SEAFOOD

DAIRY PRODUCTS

PANTRY ITEMS

FROZEN / OTHER

Weekly Meal Planner

Week of: _____

	Breakfast	Lunch	Dinner	Snack	Notes
Monday	TOTAL Carbs Fat Protein Cals	TOTAL Carbs Fat Protein Cals	TOTAL Carbs Fat Protein Cals	TOTAL Carbs Fat Protein Cals	
Tuesday	TOTAL Carbs Fat Protein Cals	TOTAL Carbs Fat Protein Cals	TOTAL Carbs Fat Protein Cals	TOTAL Carbs Fat Protein Cals	
Wednesday	TOTAL Carbs Fat Protein Cals	TOTAL Carbs Fat Protein Cals	TOTAL Carbs Fat Protein Cals	TOTAL Carbs Fat Protein Cals	
Thursday	TOTAL Carbs Fat Protein Cals	TOTAL Carbs Fat Protein Cals	TOTAL Carbs Fat Protein Cals	TOTAL Carbs Fat Protein Cals	
Friday	TOTAL Carbs Fat Protein Cals	TOTAL Carbs Fat Protein Cals	TOTAL Carbs Fat Protein Cals	TOTAL Carbs Fat Protein Cals	
Saturday	TOTAL Carbs Fat Protein Cals	TOTAL Carbs Fat Protein Cals	TOTAL Carbs Fat Protein Cals	TOTAL Carbs Fat Protein Cals	
Sunday	TOTAL Carbs Fat Protein Cals	TOTAL Carbs Fat Protein Cals	TOTAL Carbs Fat Protein Cals	TOTAL Carbs Fat Protein Cals	

Keto Grocery Inventory

DATE: _____

QTY	PRODUCE

QTY	MEAT & FISH

QTY	FROZEN FOODS

QTY	DAIRY

QTY	PANTRY

QTY	OTHER/MISC.

Low Carb Grocery Ideas

FRESH PRODUCE

☐	Asparagus	☐	Cauliflower	☐	Onions
☐	Avocado	☐	Celery	☐	Radishes
☐	Bell Peppers	☐	Cucumber	☐	Salad Mix
☐	Berries	☐	Eggplant	☐	Squash
☐	Broccoli	☐	Fennel	☐	Tomatoes
☐	Brussel Sprouts	☐	Garlic	☐	Bok Choi
☐	Cabbage	☐	Green Beans	☐	Chives
☐	Carrots	☐	Mushrooms	☐	Spinach

MEAT AND SEAFOOD

☐	Bacon	☐	Lamb	☐	Fish
☐	Beef	☐	Pork	☐	Crab
☐	Bison	☐	Rotisserie Chicken	☐	Lobster
☐	Chicken	☐	Sausage	☐	Scallops
☐	Deli meat	☐	Turkey	☐	Shrimp
☐	Ground Beef / Ground Turkey	☐	Oyster	☐	Mussels

DAIRY PRODUCTS

☐	Butter	☐	Eggs	☐	Sour Cream
☐	Cheese	☐	Greek Yogurt, full fat	☐	Ghee
☐	Cream Cheese	☐	Heavy Whipping Cream	☐	Mayo

PANTRY ITEMS

☐	Avocado oil	☐	Tea/Coffee	☐	Moon Cheese
☐	Beef Jerky	☐	Pork Rinds	☐	Low Carb Protein Bars
☐	Bone Broth	☐	Mayonnaise	☐	All Natural Peanut Butter
☐	Tuna, Salmon (canned)	☐	Low Carb Salad Dressing	☐	Stevia
☐	Coconut Butter	☐	Olive oil, extra virgin	☐	Almonds
☐	Coconut Oil	☐	Olives	☐	Spices
☐	Almond Milk	☐	Sweeteners	☐	Almond Flour

FROZEN / OTHER

☐		☐		☐	
☐		☐		☐	
☐		☐		☐	
☐		☐		☐	

Low Carb Shopping List

FRESH PRODUCE

MEAT AND SEAFOOD

DAIRY PRODUCTS

PANTRY ITEMS

FROZEN / OTHER

Weekly Meal Planner

Week of: _____

	Breakfast	Lunch	Dinner	Snack	Notes
Monday	Carbs Fat Protein Cals	Carbs Fat Protein Cals	Carbs Fat Protein Cals	Carbs Fat Protein Cals	
Tuesday	Carbs Fat Protein Cals	Carbs Fat Protein Cals	Carbs Fat Protein Cals	Carbs Fat Protein Cals	
Wednesday	Carbs Fat Protein Cals	Carbs Fat Protein Cals	Carbs Fat Protein Cals	Carbs Fat Protein Cals	
Thursday	Carbs Fat Protein Cals	Carbs Fat Protein Cals	Carbs Fat Protein Cals	Carbs Fat Protein Cals	
Friday	Carbs Fat Protein Cals	Carbs Fat Protein Cals	Carbs Fat Protein Cals	Carbs Fat Protein Cals	
Saturday	Carbs Fat Protein Cals	Carbs Fat Protein Cals	Carbs Fat Protein Cals	Carbs Fat Protein Cals	
Sunday	Carbs Fat Protein Cals	Carbs Fat Protein Cals	Carbs Fat Protein Cals	Carbs Fat Protein Cals	

Keto Grocery Inventory

DATE:

QTY	PRODUCE

QTY	MEAT & FISH

QTY	FROZEN FOODS

QTY	DAIRY

QTY	PANTRY

QTY	OTHER/MISC.

Low Carb Grocery Ideas

FRESH PRODUCE

Asparagus	Cauliflower	Onions
Avocado	Celery	Radishes
Bell Peppers	Cucumber	Salad Mix
Berries	Eggplant	Squash
Broccoli	Fennel	Tomatoes
Brussel Sprouts	Garlic	Bok Choi
Cabbage	Green Beans	Chives
Carrots	Mushrooms	Spinach

MEAT AND SEAFOOD

Bacon	Lamb	Fish
Beef	Pork	Crab
Bison	Rotisserie Chicken	Lobster
Chicken	Sausage	Scallops
Deli meat	Turkey	Shrimp
Ground Beef / Ground Turkey	Oyster	Mussels

DAIRY PRODUCTS

Butter	Eggs	Sour Cream
Cheese	Greek Yogurt, full fat	Ghee
Cream Cheese	Heavy Whipping Cream	Mayo

PANTRY ITEMS

Avocado oil	Tea/Coffee	Moon Cheese
Beef Jerky	Pork Rinds	Low Carb Protein Bars
Bone Broth	Mayonnaise	All Natural Peanut Butter
Tuna, Salmon (canned)	Low Carb Salad Dressing	Stevia
Coconut Butter	Olive oil, extra virgin	Almonds
Coconut Oil	Olives	Spices
Almond Milk	Sweeteners	Almond Flour

FROZEN / OTHER

Low Carb Shopping List

FRESH PRODUCE

MEAT AND SEAFOOD

DAIRY PRODUCTS

PANTRY ITEMS

FROZEN / OTHER

Weekly Meal Planner

Week of: _____

	Breakfast	Lunch	Dinner	Snack	Notes
Monday	TOTAL Carbs Fat Protein Cals	TOTAL Carbs Fat Protein Cals	TOTAL Carbs Fat Protein Cals	TOTAL Carbs Fat Protein Cals	
Tuesday	TOTAL Carbs Fat Protein Cals	TOTAL Carbs Fat Protein Cals	TOTAL Carbs Fat Protein Cals	TOTAL Carbs Fat Protein Cals	
Wednesday	TOTAL Carbs Fat Protein Cals	TOTAL Carbs Fat Protein Cals	TOTAL Carbs Fat Protein Cals	TOTAL Carbs Fat Protein Cals	
Thursday	TOTAL Carbs Fat Protein Cals	TOTAL Carbs Fat Protein Cals	TOTAL Carbs Fat Protein Cals	TOTAL Carbs Fat Protein Cals	
Friday	TOTAL Carbs Fat Protein Cals	TOTAL Carbs Fat Protein Cals	TOTAL Carbs Fat Protein Cals	TOTAL Carbs Fat Protein Cals	
Saturday	TOTAL Carbs Fat Protein Cals	TOTAL Carbs Fat Protein Cals	TOTAL Carbs Fat Protein Cals	TOTAL Carbs Fat Protein Cals	
Sunday	TOTAL Carbs Fat Protein Cals	TOTAL Carbs Fat Protein Cals	TOTAL Carbs Fat Protein Cals	TOTAL Carbs Fat Protein Cals	

Keto Grocery Inventory

DATE: _____

QTY	PRODUCE

QTY	MEAT & FISH

QTY	FROZEN FOODS

QTY	DAIRY

QTY	PANTRY

QTY	OTHER/MISC.

Low Carb Grocery Ideas

FRESH PRODUCE

☐	Asparagus	☐	Cauliflower	☐	Onions
☐	Avocado	☐	Celery	☐	Radishes
☐	Bell Peppers	☐	Cucumber	☐	Salad Mix
☐	Berries	☐	Eggplant	☐	Squash
☐	Broccoli	☐	Fennel	☐	Tomatoes
☐	Brussel Sprouts	☐	Garlic	☐	Bok Choi
☐	Cabbage	☐	Green Beans	☐	Chives
☐	Carrots	☐	Mushrooms	☐	Spinach

MEAT AND SEAFOOD

☐	Bacon	☐	Lamb	☐	Fish
☐	Beef	☐	Pork	☐	Crab
☐	Bison	☐	Rotisserie Chicken	☐	Lobster
☐	Chicken	☐	Sausage	☐	Scallops
☐	Deli meat	☐	Turkey	☐	Shrimp
☐	Ground Beef / Ground Turkey	☐	Oyster	☐	Mussels

DAIRY PRODUCTS

☐	Butter	☐	Eggs	☐	Sour Cream
☐	Cheese	☐	Greek Yogurt, full fat	☐	Ghee
☐	Cream Cheese	☐	Heavy Whipping Cream	☐	Mayo

PANTRY ITEMS

☐	Avocado oil	☐	Tea/Coffee	☐	Moon Cheese
☐	Beef Jerky	☐	Pork Rinds	☐	Low Carb Protein Bars
☐	Bone Broth	☐	Mayonnaise	☐	All Natural Peanut Butter
☐	Tuna, Salmon (canned)	☐	Low Carb Salad Dressing	☐	Stevia
☐	Coconut Butter	☐	Olive oil, extra virgin	☐	Almonds
☐	Coconut Oil	☐	Olives	☐	Spices
☐	Almond Milk	☐	Sweeteners	☐	Almond Flour

FROZEN / OTHER

☐		☐		☐	
☐		☐		☐	
☐		☐		☐	
☐		☐		☐	

Low Carb Shopping List

FRESH PRODUCE

MEAT AND SEAFOOD

DAIRY PRODUCTS

PANTRY ITEMS

FROZEN / OTHER

Weekly Meal Planner

Week of: _____

	Breakfast	Lunch	Dinner	Snack	Notes
Monday	TOTAL Carbs Fat Protein Cals	TOTAL Carbs Fat Protein Cals	TOTAL Carbs Fat Protein Cals	TOTAL Carbs Fat Protein Cals	
Tuesday	TOTAL Carbs Fat Protein Cals	TOTAL Carbs Fat Protein Cals	TOTAL Carbs Fat Protein Cals	TOTAL Carbs Fat Protein Cals	
Wednesday	TOTAL Carbs Fat Protein Cals	TOTAL Carbs Fat Protein Cals	TOTAL Carbs Fat Protein Cals	TOTAL Carbs Fat Protein Cals	
Thursday	TOTAL Carbs Fat Protein Cals	TOTAL Carbs Fat Protein Cals	TOTAL Carbs Fat Protein Cals	TOTAL Carbs Fat Protein Cals	
Friday	TOTAL Carbs Fat Protein Cals	TOTAL Carbs Fat Protein Cals	TOTAL Carbs Fat Protein Cals	TOTAL Carbs Fat Protein Cals	
Saturday	TOTAL Carbs Fat Protein Cals	TOTAL Carbs Fat Protein Cals	TOTAL Carbs Fat Protein Cals	TOTAL Carbs Fat Protein Cals	
Sunday	TOTAL Carbs Fat Protein Cals	TOTAL Carbs Fat Protein Cals	TOTAL Carbs Fat Protein Cals	TOTAL Carbs Fat Protein Cals	

Keto Grocery Inventory

DATE: _____

QTY	PRODUCE

QTY	MEAT & FISH

QTY	FROZEN FOODS

QTY	DAIRY

QTY	PANTRY

QTY	OTHER/MISC.

Low Carb Grocery Ideas

FRESH PRODUCE

Asparagus	Cauliflower	Onions
Avocado	Celery	Radishes
Bell Peppers	Cucumber	Salad Mix
Berries	Eggplant	Squash
Broccoli	Fennel	Tomatoes
Brussel Sprouts	Garlic	Bok Choi
Cabbage	Green Beans	Chives
Carrots	Mushrooms	Spinach

MEAT AND SEAFOOD

Bacon	Lamb	Fish
Beef	Pork	Crab
Bison	Rotisserie Chicken	Lobster
Chicken	Sausage	Scallops
Deli meat	Turkey	Shrimp
Ground Beef / Ground Turkey	Oyster	Mussels

DAIRY PRODUCTS

Butter	Eggs	Sour Cream
Cheese	Greek Yogurt, full fat	Ghee
Cream Cheese	Heavy Whipping Cream	Mayo

PANTRY ITEMS

Avocado oil	Tea/Coffee	Moon Cheese
Beef Jerky	Pork Rinds	Low Carb Protein Bars
Bone Broth	Mayonnaise	All Natural Peanut Butter
Tuna, Salmon (canned)	Low Carb Salad Dressing	Stevia
Coconut Butter	Olive oil, extra virgin	Almonds
Coconut Oil	Olives	Spices
Almond Milk	Sweeteners	Almond Flour

FROZEN / OTHER

Low Carb Shopping List

FRESH PRODUCE

MEAT AND SEAFOOD

DAIRY PRODUCTS

PANTRY ITEMS

FROZEN / OTHER

Weekly Meal Planner

Week of: _____

	Breakfast	Lunch	Dinner	Snack	Notes
Monday	Carbs Fat Protein TOTAL Cals	Carbs Fat Protein TOTAL Cals	Carbs Fat Protein TOTAL Cals	Carbs Fat Protein TOTAL Cals	
Tuesday	Carbs Fat Protein TOTAL Cals	Carbs Fat Protein TOTAL Cals	Carbs Fat Protein TOTAL Cals	Carbs Fat Protein TOTAL Cals	
Wednesday	Carbs Fat Protein TOTAL Cals	Carbs Fat Protein TOTAL Cals	Carbs Fat Protein TOTAL Cals	Carbs Fat Protein TOTAL Cals	
Thursday	Carbs Fat Protein TOTAL Cals	Carbs Fat Protein TOTAL Cals	Carbs Fat Protein TOTAL Cals	Carbs Fat Protein TOTAL Cals	
Friday	Carbs Fat Protein TOTAL Cals	Carbs Fat Protein TOTAL Cals	Carbs Fat Protein TOTAL Cals	Carbs Fat Protein TOTAL Cals	
Saturday	Carbs Fat Protein TOTAL Cals	Carbs Fat Protein TOTAL Cals	Carbs Fat Protein TOTAL Cals	Carbs Fat Protein TOTAL Cals	
Sunday	Carbs Fat Protein TOTAL Cals	Carbs Fat Protein TOTAL Cals	Carbs Fat Protein TOTAL Cals	Carbs Fat Protein TOTAL Cals	

Keto Grocery Inventory

DATE: _____

QTY	PRODUCE

QTY	MEAT & FISH

QTY	FROZEN FOODS

QTY	DAIRY

QTY	PANTRY

QTY	OTHER/MISC.

Low Carb Grocery Ideas

FRESH PRODUCE

Asparagus	Cauliflower	Onions
Avocado	Celery	Radishes
Bell Peppers	Cucumber	Salad Mix
Berries	Eggplant	Squash
Broccoli	Fennel	Tomatoes
Brussel Sprouts	Garlic	Bok Choi
Cabbage	Green Beans	Chives
Carrots	Mushrooms	Spinach

MEAT AND SEAFOOD

Bacon	Lamb	Fish
Beef	Pork	Crab
Bison	Rotisserie Chicken	Lobster
Chicken	Sausage	Scallops
Deli meat	Turkey	Shrimp
Ground Beef / Ground Turkey	Oyster	Mussels

DAIRY PRODUCTS

Butter	Eggs	Sour Cream
Cheese	Greek Yogurt, full fat	Ghee
Cream Cheese	Heavy Whipping Cream	Mayo

PANTRY ITEMS

Avocado oil	Tea/Coffee	Moon Cheese
Beef Jerky	Pork Rinds	Low Carb Protein Bars
Bone Broth	Mayonnaise	All Natural Peanut Butter
Tuna, Salmon (canned)	Low Carb Salad Dressing	Stevia
Coconut Butter	Olive oil, extra virgin	Almonds
Coconut Oil	Olives	Spices
Almond Milk	Sweeteners	Almond Flour

FROZEN / OTHER

Low Carb Shopping List

FRESH PRODUCE

MEAT AND SEAFOOD

DAIRY PRODUCTS

PANTRY ITEMS

FROZEN / OTHER

Weekly Meal Planner

Week of: _____

	Breakfast	Lunch	Dinner	Snack	Notes
Monday	TOTAL Carbs Fat Protein Cals	TOTAL Carbs Fat Protein Cals	TOTAL Carbs Fat Protein Cals	TOTAL Carbs Fat Protein Cals	
Tuesday	TOTAL Carbs Fat Protein Cals	TOTAL Carbs Fat Protein Cals	TOTAL Carbs Fat Protein Cals	TOTAL Carbs Fat Protein Cals	
Wednesday	TOTAL Carbs Fat Protein Cals	TOTAL Carbs Fat Protein Cals	TOTAL Carbs Fat Protein Cals	TOTAL Carbs Fat Protein Cals	
Thursday	TOTAL Carbs Fat Protein Cals	TOTAL Carbs Fat Protein Cals	TOTAL Carbs Fat Protein Cals	TOTAL Carbs Fat Protein Cals	
Friday	TOTAL Carbs Fat Protein Cals	TOTAL Carbs Fat Protein Cals	TOTAL Carbs Fat Protein Cals	TOTAL Carbs Fat Protein Cals	
Saturday	TOTAL Carbs Fat Protein Cals	TOTAL Carbs Fat Protein Cals	TOTAL Carbs Fat Protein Cals	TOTAL Carbs Fat Protein Cals	
Sunday	TOTAL Carbs Fat Protein Cals	TOTAL Carbs Fat Protein Cals	TOTAL Carbs Fat Protein Cals	TOTAL Carbs Fat Protein Cals	

Keto Grocery Inventory

DATE: _____

QTY	PRODUCE

QTY	MEAT & FISH

QTY	FROZEN FOODS

QTY	DAIRY

QTY	PANTRY

QTY	OTHER/MISC.

Low Carb Grocery Ideas

FRESH PRODUCE

☐ Asparagus	☐ Cauliflower	☐ Onions
☐ Avocado	☐ Celery	☐ Radishes
☐ Bell Peppers	☐ Cucumber	☐ Salad Mix
☐ Berries	☐ Eggplant	☐ Squash
☐ Broccoli	☐ Fennel	☐ Tomatoes
☐ Brussel Sprouts	☐ Garlic	☐ Bok Choi
☐ Cabbage	☐ Green Beans	☐ Chives
☐ Carrots	☐ Mushrooms	☐ Spinach

MEAT AND SEAFOOD

☐ Bacon	☐ Lamb	☐ Fish
☐ Beef	☐ Pork	☐ Crab
☐ Bison	☐ Rotisserie Chicken	☐ Lobster
☐ Chicken	☐ Sausage	☐ Scallops
☐ Deli meat	☐ Turkey	☐ Shrimp
☐ Ground Beef / Ground Turkey	☐ Oyster	☐ Mussels

DAIRY PRODUCTS

☐ Butter	☐ Eggs	☐ Sour Cream
☐ Cheese	☐ Greek Yogurt, full fat	☐ Ghee
☐ Cream Cheese	☐ Heavy Whipping Cream	☐ Mayo

PANTRY ITEMS

☐ Avocado oil	☐ Tea/Coffee	☐ Moon Cheese
☐ Beef Jerky	☐ Pork Rinds	☐ Low Carb Protein Bars
☐ Bone Broth	☐ Mayonnaise	☐ All Natural Peanut Butter
☐ Tuna, Salmon (canned)	☐ Low Carb Salad Dressing	☐ Stevia
☐ Coconut Butter	☐ Olive oil, extra virgin	☐ Almonds
☐ Coconut Oil	☐ Olives	☐ Spices
☐ Almond Milk	☐ Sweeteners	☐ Almond Flour

FROZEN / OTHER

☐	☐	☐
☐	☐	☐
☐	☐	☐
☐	☐	☐

Low Carb Shopping List

FRESH PRODUCE

MEAT AND SEAFOOD

DAIRY PRODUCTS

PANTRY ITEMS

FROZEN / OTHER

Weekly Meal Planner

Week of: _____

	Breakfast	Lunch	Dinner	Snack	Notes
Monday	Carbs Fat Protein TOTAL Cals	Carbs Fat Protein TOTAL Cals	Carbs Fat Protein TOTAL Cals	Carbs Fat Protein TOTAL Cals	
Tuesday	Carbs Fat Protein TOTAL Cals	Carbs Fat Protein TOTAL Cals	Carbs Fat Protein TOTAL Cals	Carbs Fat Protein TOTAL Cals	
Wednesday	Carbs Fat Protein TOTAL Cals	Carbs Fat Protein TOTAL Cals	Carbs Fat Protein TOTAL Cals	Carbs Fat Protein TOTAL Cals	
Thursday	Carbs Fat Protein TOTAL Cals	Carbs Fat Protein TOTAL Cals	Carbs Fat Protein TOTAL Cals	Carbs Fat Protein TOTAL Cals	
Friday	Carbs Fat Protein TOTAL Cals	Carbs Fat Protein TOTAL Cals	Carbs Fat Protein TOTAL Cals	Carbs Fat Protein TOTAL Cals	
Saturday	Carbs Fat Protein TOTAL Cals	Carbs Fat Protein TOTAL Cals	Carbs Fat Protein TOTAL Cals	Carbs Fat Protein TOTAL Cals	
Sunday	Carbs Fat Protein TOTAL Cals	Carbs Fat Protein TOTAL Cals	Carbs Fat Protein TOTAL Cals	Carbs Fat Protein TOTAL Cals	

Keto Grocery Inventory

DATE: _____

QTY	PRODUCE

QTY	MEAT & FISH

QTY	FROZEN FOODS

QTY	DAIRY

QTY	PANTRY

QTY	OTHER/MISC.

Low Carb Grocery Ideas

FRESH PRODUCE

☐ Asparagus	☐ Cauliflower	☐ Onions
☐ Avocado	☐ Celery	☐ Radishes
☐ Bell Peppers	☐ Cucumber	☐ Salad Mix
☐ Berries	☐ Eggplant	☐ Squash
☐ Broccoli	☐ Fennel	☐ Tomatoes
☐ Brussel Sprouts	☐ Garlic	☐ Bok Choi
☐ Cabbage	☐ Green Beans	☐ Chives
☐ Carrots	☐ Mushrooms	☐ Spinach

MEAT AND SEAFOOD

☐ Bacon	☐ Lamb	☐ Fish
☐ Beef	☐ Pork	☐ Crab
☐ Bison	☐ Rotisserie Chicken	☐ Lobster
☐ Chicken	☐ Sausage	☐ Scallops
☐ Deli meat	☐ Turkey	☐ Shrimp
☐ Ground Beef / Ground Turkey	☐ Oyster	☐ Mussels

DAIRY PRODUCTS

☐ Butter	☐ Eggs	☐ Sour Cream
☐ Cheese	☐ Greek Yogurt, full fat	☐ Ghee
☐ Cream Cheese	☐ Heavy Whipping Cream	☐ Mayo

PANTRY ITEMS

☐ Avocado oil	☐ Tea/Coffee	☐ Moon Cheese
☐ Beef Jerky	☐ Pork Rinds	☐ Low Carb Protein Bars
☐ Bone Broth	☐ Mayonnaise	☐ All Natural Peanut Butter
☐ Tuna, Salmon (canned)	☐ Low Carb Salad Dressing	☐ Stevia
☐ Coconut Butter	☐ Olive oil, extra virgin	☐ Almonds
☐ Coconut Oil	☐ Olives	☐ Spices
☐ Almond Milk	☐ Sweeteners	☐ Almond Flour

FROZEN / OTHER

☐	☐	☐
☐	☐	☐
☐	☐	☐
☐	☐	☐

Low Carb Shopping List

FRESH PRODUCE

MEAT AND SEAFOOD

DAIRY PRODUCTS

PANTRY ITEMS

FROZEN / OTHER

Weekly Meal Planner

Week of: _____

	Breakfast	Lunch	Dinner	Snack	Notes
Monday	Carbs Fat Protein TOTAL Cals	Carbs Fat Protein TOTAL Cals	Carbs Fat Protein TOTAL Cals	Carbs Fat Protein TOTAL Cals	
Tuesday	Carbs Fat Protein TOTAL Cals	Carbs Fat Protein TOTAL Cals	Carbs Fat Protein TOTAL Cals	Carbs Fat Protein TOTAL Cals	
Wednesday	Carbs Fat Protein TOTAL Cals	Carbs Fat Protein TOTAL Cals	Carbs Fat Protein TOTAL Cals	Carbs Fat Protein TOTAL Cals	
Thursday	Carbs Fat Protein TOTAL Cals	Carbs Fat Protein TOTAL Cals	Carbs Fat Protein TOTAL Cals	Carbs Fat Protein TOTAL Cals	
Friday	Carbs Fat Protein TOTAL Cals	Carbs Fat Protein TOTAL Cals	Carbs Fat Protein TOTAL Cals	Carbs Fat Protein TOTAL Cals	
Saturday	Carbs Fat Protein TOTAL Cals	Carbs Fat Protein TOTAL Cals	Carbs Fat Protein TOTAL Cals	Carbs Fat Protein TOTAL Cals	
Sunday	Carbs Fat Protein TOTAL Cals	Carbs Fat Protein TOTAL Cals	Carbs Fat Protein TOTAL Cals	Carbs Fat Protein TOTAL Cals	

Keto Grocery Inventory

DATE: _____

QTY	PRODUCE

QTY	MEAT & FISH

QTY	FROZEN FOODS

QTY	DAIRY

QTY	PANTRY

QTY	OTHER/MISC.

Low Carb Grocery Ideas

FRESH PRODUCE

☐ Asparagus	☐ Cauliflower	☐ Onions
☐ Avocado	☐ Celery	☐ Radishes
☐ Bell Peppers	☐ Cucumber	☐ Salad Mix
☐ Berries	☐ Eggplant	☐ Squash
☐ Broccoli	☐ Fennel	☐ Tomatoes
☐ Brussel Sprouts	☐ Garlic	☐ Bok Choi
☐ Cabbage	☐ Green Beans	☐ Chives
☐ Carrots	☐ Mushrooms	☐ Spinach

MEAT AND SEAFOOD

☐ Bacon	☐ Lamb	☐ Fish
☐ Beef	☐ Pork	☐ Crab
☐ Bison	☐ Rotisserie Chicken	☐ Lobster
☐ Chicken	☐ Sausage	☐ Scallops
☐ Deli meat	☐ Turkey	☐ Shrimp
☐ Ground Beef / Ground Turkey	☐ Oyster	☐ Mussels

DAIRY PRODUCTS

☐ Butter	☐ Eggs	☐ Sour Cream
☐ Cheese	☐ Greek Yogurt, full fat	☐ Ghee
☐ Cream Cheese	☐ Heavy Whipping Cream	☐ Mayo

PANTRY ITEMS

☐ Avocado oil	☐ Tea/Coffee	☐ Moon Cheese
☐ Beef Jerky	☐ Pork Rinds	☐ Low Carb Protein Bars
☐ Bone Broth	☐ Mayonnaise	☐ All Natural Peanut Butter
☐ Tuna, Salmon (canned)	☐ Low Carb Salad Dressing	☐ Stevia
☐ Coconut Butter	☐ Olive oil, extra virgin	☐ Almonds
☐ Coconut Oil	☐ Olives	☐ Spices
☐ Almond Milk	☐ Sweeteners	☐ Almond Flour

FROZEN / OTHER

☐	☐	☐
☐	☐	☐
☐	☐	☐
☐	☐	☐

Low Carb Shopping List

FRESH PRODUCE

MEAT AND SEAFOOD

DAIRY PRODUCTS

PANTRY ITEMS

FROZEN / OTHER

Weekly Meal Planner

Week of: _____

	Breakfast	Lunch	Dinner	Snack	Notes
Monday	Carb: Fat Protein TOTAL Cals	Carb: Fat Protein TOTAL Cals	Carb: Fat Protein TOTAL Cals	Carb: Fat Protein TOTAL Cals	___ ___ ___
Tuesday	Carb: Fat Protein TOTAL Cals	Carb: Fat Protein TOTAL Cals	Carb: Fat Protein TOTAL Cals	Carb: Fat Protein TOTAL Cals	___ ___ ___
Wednesday	Carb: Fat Protein TOTAL Cals	Carb: Fat Protein TOTAL Cals	Carb: Fat Protein TOTAL Cals	Carb: Fat Protein TOTAL Cals	___ ___ ___
Thursday	Carb: Fat Protein TOTAL Cals	Carb: Fat Protein TOTAL Cals	Carb: Fat Protein TOTAL Cals	Carb: Fat Protein TOTAL Cals	___ ___ ___
Friday	Carb: Fat Protein TOTAL Cals	Carb: Fat Protein TOTAL Cals	Carb: Fat Protein TOTAL Cals	Carb: Fat Protein TOTAL Cals	___ ___ ___
Saturday	Carb: Fat Protein TOTAL Cals	Carb: Fat Protein TOTAL Cals	Carb: Fat Protein TOTAL Cals	Carb: Fat Protein TOTAL Cals	___ ___ ___
Sunday	Carb: Fat Protein TOTAL Cals	Carb: Fat Protein TOTAL Cals	Carb: Fat Protein TOTAL Cals	Carb: Fat Protein TOTAL Cals	___ ___ ___

Keto Grocery Inventory

DATE: _____

QTY	PRODUCE

QTY	MEAT & FISH

QTY	FROZEN FOODS

QTY	DAIRY

QTY	PANTRY

QTY	OTHER/MISC.

Low Carb Grocery Ideas

FRESH PRODUCE

☐	Asparagus	☐	Cauliflower	☐	Onions
☐	Avocado	☐	Celery	☐	Radishes
☐	Bell Peppers	☐	Cucumber	☐	Salad Mix
☐	Berries	☐	Eggplant	☐	Squash
☐	Broccoli	☐	Fennel	☐	Tomatoes
☐	Brussel Sprouts	☐	Garlic	☐	Bok Choi
☐	Cabbage	☐	Green Beans	☐	Chives
☐	Carrots	☐	Mushrooms	☐	Spinach

MEAT AND SEAFOOD

☐	Bacon	☐	Lamb	☐	Fish
☐	Beef	☐	Pork	☐	Crab
☐	Bison	☐	Rotisserie Chicken	☐	Lobster
☐	Chicken	☐	Sausage	☐	Scallops
☐	Deli meat	☐	Turkey	☐	Shrimp
☐	Ground Beef / Ground Turkey	☐	Oyster	☐	Mussels

DAIRY PRODUCTS

☐	Butter	☐	Eggs	☐	Sour Cream
☐	Cheese	☐	Greek Yogurt, full fat	☐	Ghee
☐	Cream Cheese	☐	Heavy Whipping Cream	☐	Mayo

PANTRY ITEMS

☐	Avocado oil	☐	Tea/Coffee	☐	Moon Cheese
☐	Beef Jerky	☐	Pork Rinds	☐	Low Carb Protein Bars
☐	Bone Broth	☐	Mayonnaise	☐	All Natural Peanut Butter
☐	Tuna, Salmon (canned)	☐	Low Carb Salad Dressing	☐	Stevia
☐	Coconut Butter	☐	Olive oil, extra virgin	☐	Almonds
☐	Coconut Oil	☐	Olives	☐	Spices
☐	Almond Milk	☐	Sweeteners	☐	Almond Flour

FROZEN / OTHER

☐		☐		☐	
☐		☐		☐	
☐		☐		☐	
☐		☐		☐	

Low Carb Shopping List

FRESH PRODUCE

MEAT AND SEAFOOD

DAIRY PRODUCTS

PANTRY ITEMS

FROZEN / OTHER

Weekly Meal Planner

Week of: _____

	Breakfast	Lunch	Dinner	Snack	Notes
Monday	TOTAL Carbs Fat Protein Cals	TOTAL Carbs Fat Protein Cals	TOTAL Carbs Fat Protein Cals	TOTAL Carbs Fat Protein Cals	
Tuesday	TOTAL Carbs Fat Protein Cals	TOTAL Carbs Fat Protein Cals	TOTAL Carbs Fat Protein Cals	TOTAL Carbs Fat Protein Cals	
Wednesday	TOTAL Carbs Fa Protein Cals	TOTAL Carbs Fat Protein Cals	TOTAL Carbs Fat Protein Cals	TOTAL Carbs Fat Protein Cals	
Thursday	TOTAL Carbs Fa Protein Cals	TOTAL Carbs Fat Protein Cals	TOTAL Carbs Fat Protein Cals	TOTAL Carbs Fat Protein Cals	
Friday	TOTAL Carbs Fa Protein Cals	TOTAL Carbs Fat Protein Cals	TOTAL Carbs Fat Protein Cals	TOTAL Carbs Fat Protein Cals	
Saturday	TOTAL Carbs Fa Protein Cals	TOTAL Carbs Fat Protein Cals	TOTAL Carbs Fat Protein Cals	TOTAL Carbs Fat Protein Cals	
Sunday	TOTAL Carbs Fa Protein Cals	TOTAL Carbs Fat Protein Cals	TOTAL Carbs Fat Protein Cals	TOTAL Carbs Fat Protein Cals	

Keto Grocery Inventory

DATE: _____

QTY	PRODUCE

QTY	MEAT & FISH

QTY	FROZEN FOODS

QTY	DAIRY

QTY	PANTRY

QTY	OTHER/MISC.

Low Carb Grocery Ideas

FRESH PRODUCE

Asparagus	Cauliflower	Onions
Avocado	Celery	Radishes
Bell Peppers	Cucumber	Salad Mix
Berries	Eggplant	Squash
Broccoli	Fennel	Tomatoes
Brussel Sprouts	Garlic	Bok Choi
Cabbage	Green Beans	Chives
Carrots	Mushrooms	Spinach

MEAT AND SEAFOOD

Bacon	Lamb	Fish
Beef	Pork	Crab
Bison	Rotisserie Chicken	Lobster
Chicken	Sausage	Scallops
Deli meat	Turkey	Shrimp
Ground Beef / Ground Turkey	Oyster	Mussels

DAIRY PRODUCTS

Butter	Eggs	Sour Cream
Cheese	Greek Yogurt, full fat	Ghee
Cream Cheese	Heavy Whipping Cream	Mayo

PANTRY ITEMS

Avocado oil	Tea/Coffee	Moon Cheese
Beef Jerky	Pork Rinds	Low Carb Protein Bars
Bone Broth	Mayonnaise	All Natural Peanut Butter
Tuna, Salmon (canned)	Low Carb Salad Dressing	Stevia
Coconut Butter	Olive oil, extra virgin	Almonds
Coconut Oil	Olives	Spices
Almond Milk	Sweeteners	Almond Flour

FROZEN / OTHER

Low Carb Shopping List

FRESH PRODUCE

MEAT AND SEAFOOD

DAIRY PRODUCTS

PANTRY ITEMS

FROZEN / OTHER

Weekly Meal Planner

Week of: _____

	Breakfast	Lunch	Dinner	Snack	Notes
Monday					_____
	TOTAL Carbs Fat Protein Cals	TOTAL Carbs Fat Protein Cals	TOTAL Carbs Fat Protein Cals	TOTAL Carbs Fat Protein Cals	_____
Tuesday					_____
	TOTAL Carbs Fat Protein Cals	TOTAL Carbs Fat Protein Cals	TOTAL Carbs Fat Protein Cals	TOTAL Carbs Fat Protein Cals	_____
Wednesday					_____
	TOTAL Carbs Fat Protein Cals	TOTAL Carbs Fat Protein Cals	TOTAL Carbs Fat Protein Cals	TOTAL Carbs Fat Protein Cals	_____
Thursday					_____
	TOTAL Carbs Fat Protein Cals	TOTAL Carbs Fat Protein Cals	TOTAL Carbs Fat Protein Cals	TOTAL Carbs Fat Protein Cals	_____
Friday					_____
	TOTAL Carbs Fat Protein Cals	TOTAL Carbs Fat Protein Cals	TOTAL Carbs Fat Protein Cals	TOTAL Carbs Fat Protein Cals	_____
Saturday					_____
	TOTAL Carbs Fat Protein Cals	TOTAL Carbs Fat Protein Cals	TOTAL Carbs Fat Protein Cals	TOTAL Carbs Fat Protein Cals	_____
Sunday					_____
	TOTAL Carbs Fat Protein Cals	TOTAL Carbs Fat Protein Cals	TOTAL Carbs Fat Protein Cals	TOTAL Carbs Fat Protein Cals	_____

Keto Grocery Inventory

DATE: _____

QTY	PRODUCE

QTY	MEAT & FISH

QTY	FROZEN FOODS

QTY	DAIRY

QTY	PANTRY

QTY	OTHER/MISC.

Low Carb Grocery Ideas

FRESH PRODUCE

☐	Asparagus	☐	Cauliflower	☐	Onions
☐	Avocado	☐	Celery	☐	Radishes
☐	Bell Peppers	☐	Cucumber	☐	Salad Mix
☐	Berries	☐	Eggplant	☐	Squash
☐	Broccoli	☐	Fennel	☐	Tomatoes
☐	Brussel Sprouts	☐	Garlic	☐	Bok Choi
☐	Cabbage	☐	Green Beans	☐	Chives
☐	Carrots	☐	Mushrooms	☐	Spinach

MEAT AND SEAFOOD

☐	Bacon	☐	Lamb	☐	Fish
☐	Beef	☐	Pork	☐	Crab
☐	Bison	☐	Rotisserie Chicken	☐	Lobster
☐	Chicken	☐	Sausage	☐	Scallops
☐	Deli meat	☐	Turkey	☐	Shrimp
☐	Ground Beef / Ground Turkey	☐	Oyster	☐	Mussels

DAIRY PRODUCTS

☐	Butter	☐	Eggs	☐	Sour Cream
☐	Cheese	☐	Greek Yogurt, full fat	☐	Ghee
☐	Cream Cheese	☐	Heavy Whipping Cream	☐	Mayo

PANTRY ITEMS

☐	Avocado oil	☐	Tea/Coffee	☐	Moon Cheese
☐	Beef Jerky	☐	Pork Rinds	☐	Low Carb Protein Bars
☐	Bone Broth	☐	Mayonnaise	☐	All Natural Peanut Butter
☐	Tuna, Salmon (canned)	☐	Low Carb Salad Dressing	☐	Stevia
☐	Coconut Butter	☐	Olive oil, extra virgin	☐	Almonds
☐	Coconut Oil	☐	Olives	☐	Spices
☐	Almond Milk	☐	Sweeteners	☐	Almond Flour

FROZEN / OTHER

☐		☐		☐	
☐		☐		☐	
☐		☐		☐	
☐		☐		☐	

Low Carb Shopping List

FRESH PRODUCE

MEAT AND SEAFOOD

DAIRY PRODUCTS

PANTRY ITEMS

FROZEN / OTHER

Weekly Meal Planner

Week of: _____

	Breakfast	Lunch	Dinner	Snack	Notes
Monday	TOTAL Carbs Fat Protein Cals	TOTAL Carbs Fat Protein Cals	TOTAL Carbs Fat Protein Cals	TOTAL Carbs Fat Protein Cals	
Tuesday	TOTAL Carbs Fat Protein Cals	TOTAL Carbs Fat Protein Cals	TOTAL Carbs Fat Protein Cals	TOTAL Carbs Fat Protein Cals	
Wednesday	TOTAL Carbs Fat Protein Cals	TOTAL Carbs Fat Protein Cals	TOTAL Carbs Fat Protein Cals	TOTAL Carbs Fat Protein Cals	
Thursday	TOTAL Carbs Fat Protein Cals	TOTAL Carbs Fat Protein Cals	TOTAL Carbs Fat Protein Cals	TOTAL Carbs Fat Protein Cals	
Friday	TOTAL Carbs Fat Protein Cals	TOTAL Carbs Fat Protein Cals	TOTAL Carbs Fat Protein Cals	TOTAL Carbs Fat Protein Cals	
Saturday	TOTAL Carbs Fat Protein Cals	TOTAL Carbs Fat Protein Cals	TOTAL Carbs Fat Protein Cals	TOTAL Carbs Fat Protein Cals	
Sunday	TOTAL Carbs Fat Protein Cals	TOTAL Carbs Fat Protein Cals	TOTAL Carbs Fat Protein Cals	TOTAL Carbs Fat Protein Cals	

Keto Grocery Inventory

DATE: _____

QTY	PRODUCE

QTY	MEAT & FISH

QTY	FROZEN FOODS

QTY	DAIRY

QTY	PANTRY

QTY	OTHER/MISC.

Low Carb Grocery Ideas

FRESH PRODUCE

☐ Asparagus	☐ Cauliflower	☐ Onions
☐ Avocado	☐ Celery	☐ Radishes
☐ Bell Peppers	☐ Cucumber	☐ Salad Mix
☐ Berries	☐ Eggplant	☐ Squash
☐ Broccoli	☐ Fennel	☐ Tomatoes
☐ Brussel Sprouts	☐ Garlic	☐ Bok Choi
☐ Cabbage	☐ Green Beans	☐ Chives
☐ Carrots	☐ Mushrooms	☐ Spinach

MEAT AND SEAFOOD

☐ Bacon	☐ Lamb	☐ Fish
☐ Beef	☐ Pork	☐ Crab
☐ Bison	☐ Rotisserie Chicken	☐ Lobster
☐ Chicken	☐ Sausage	☐ Scallops
☐ Deli meat	☐ Turkey	☐ Shrimp
☐ Ground Beef / Ground Turkey	☐ Oyster	☐ Mussels

DAIRY PRODUCTS

☐ Butter	☐ Eggs	☐ Sour Cream
☐ Cheese	☐ Greek Yogurt, full fat	☐ Ghee
☐ Cream Cheese	☐ Heavy Whipping Cream	☐ Mayo

PANTRY ITEMS

☐ Avocado oil	☐ Tea/Coffee	☐ Moon Cheese
☐ Beef Jerky	☐ Pork Rinds	☐ Low Carb Protein Bars
☐ Bone Broth	☐ Mayonnaise	☐ All Natural Peanut Butter
☐ Tuna, Salmon (canned)	☐ Low Carb Salad Dressing	☐ Stevia
☐ Coconut Butter	☐ Olive oil, extra virgin	☐ Almonds
☐ Coconut Oil	☐ Olives	☐ Spices
☐ Almond Milk	☐ Sweeteners	☐ Almond Flour

FROZEN / OTHER

☐	☐	☐
☐	☐	☐
☐	☐	☐
☐	☐	☐

Low Carb Shopping List

FRESH PRODUCE

MEAT AND SEAFOOD

DAIRY PRODUCTS

PANTRY ITEMS

FROZEN / OTHER

Weekly Meal Planner

Week of: _____

	Breakfast	Lunch	Dinner	Snack	Notes
Monday	TOTAL Carbs Fat Protein Cals	TOTAL Carbs Fat Protein Cals	TOTAL Carbs Fat Protein Cals	TOTAL Carbs Fat Protein Cals	
Tuesday	TOTAL Carbs Fat Protein Cals	TOTAL Carbs Fat Protein Cals	TOTAL Carbs Fat Protein Cals	TOTAL Carbs Fat Protein Cals	
Wednesday	TOTAL Carbs Fa Protein Cals	TOTAL Carbs Fat Protein Cals	TOTAL Carbs Fat Protein Cals	TOTAL Carbs Fat Protein Cals	
Thursday	TOTAL Carbs Fa Protein Cals	TOTAL Carbs Fat Protein Cals	TOTAL Carbs Fat Protein Cals	TOTAL Carbs Fat Protein Cals	
Friday	TOTAL Carbs Fa Protein Cals	TOTAL Carbs Fat Protein Cals	TOTAL Carbs Fat Protein Cals	TOTAL Carbs Fat Protein Cals	
Saturday	TOTAL Carbs Fa Protein Cals	TOTAL Carbs Fat Protein Cals	TOTAL Carbs Fat Protein Cals	TOTAL Carbs Fat Protein Cals	
Sunday	TOTAL Carbs Fa Protein Cals	TOTAL Carbs Fat Protein Cals	TOTAL Carbs Fat Protein Cals	TOTAL Carbs Fat Protein Cals	

Keto Grocery Inventory

DATE: _____

QTY	PRODUCE

QTY	MEAT & FISH

QTY	FROZEN FOODS

QTY	DAIRY

QTY	PANTRY

QTY	OTHER/MISC.

Low Carb Grocery Ideas

FRESH PRODUCE

☐ Asparagus	☐ Cauliflower	☐ Onions
☐ Avocado	☐ Celery	☐ Radishes
☐ Bell Peppers	☐ Cucumber	☐ Salad Mix
☐ Berries	☐ Eggplant	☐ Squash
☐ Broccoli	☐ Fennel	☐ Tomatoes
☐ Brussel Sprouts	☐ Garlic	☐ Bok Choi
☐ Cabbage	☐ Green Beans	☐ Chives
☐ Carrots	☐ Mushrooms	☐ Spinach

MEAT AND SEAFOOD

☐ Bacon	☐ Lamb	☐ Fish
☐ Beef	☐ Pork	☐ Crab
☐ Bison	☐ Rotisserie Chicken	☐ Lobster
☐ Chicken	☐ Sausage	☐ Scallops
☐ Deli meat	☐ Turkey	☐ Shrimp
☐ Ground Beef / Ground Turkey	☐ Oyster	☐ Mussels

DAIRY PRODUCTS

☐ Butter	☐ Eggs	☐ Sour Cream
☐ Cheese	☐ Greek Yogurt, full fat	☐ Ghee
☐ Cream Cheese	☐ Heavy Whipping Cream	☐ Mayo

PANTRY ITEMS

☐ Avocado oil	☐ Tea/Coffee	☐ Moon Cheese
☐ Beef Jerky	☐ Pork Rinds	☐ Low Carb Protein Bars
☐ Bone Broth	☐ Mayonnaise	☐ All Natural Peanut Butter
☐ Tuna, Salmon (canned)	☐ Low Carb Salad Dressing	☐ Stevia
☐ Coconut Butter	☐ Olive oil, extra virgin	☐ Almonds
☐ Coconut Oil	☐ Olives	☐ Spices
☐ Almond Milk	☐ Sweeteners	☐ Almond Flour

FROZEN / OTHER

☐	☐	☐
☐	☐	☐
☐	☐	☐
☐	☐	☐

Low Carb Shopping List

FRESH PRODUCE

MEAT AND SEAFOOD

DAIRY PRODUCTS

PANTRY ITEMS

FROZEN / OTHER

Weekly Meal Planner

Week of: _____

	Breakfast	Lunch	Dinner	Snack	Notes
Monday	Carbs Fat Protein TOTAL Cals	Carbs Fat Protein TOTAL Cals	Carbs Fat Protein TOTAL Cals	Carbs Fat Protein TOTAL Cals	
Tuesday	Carbs Fat Protein TOTAL Cals	Carbs Fat Protein TOTAL Cals	Carbs Fat Protein TOTAL Cals	Carbs Fat Protein TOTAL Cals	
Wednesday	Carbs Fat Protein TOTAL Cals	Carbs Fat Protein TOTAL Cals	Carbs Fat Protein TOTAL Cals	Carbs Fat Protein TOTAL Cals	
Thursday	Carbs Fat Protein TOTAL Cals	Carbs Fat Protein TOTAL Cals	Carbs Fat Protein TOTAL Cals	Carbs Fat Protein TOTAL Cals	
Friday	Carbs Fat Protein TOTAL Cals	Carbs Fat Protein TOTAL Cals	Carbs Fat Protein TOTAL Cals	Carbs Fat Protein TOTAL Cals	
Saturday	Carbs Fat Protein TOTAL Cals	Carbs Fat Protein TOTAL Cals	Carbs Fat Protein TOTAL Cals	Carbs Fat Protein TOTAL Cals	
Sunday	Carbs Fat Protein TOTAL Cals	Carbs Fat Protein TOTAL Cals	Carbs Fat Protein TOTAL Cals	Carbs Fat Protein TOTAL Cals	

Keto Grocery Inventory

DATE: _____

QTY	PRODUCE

QTY	MEAT & FISH

QTY	FROZEN FOODS

QTY	DAIRY

QTY	PANTRY

QTY	OTHER/MISC.

Low Carb Grocery Ideas

FRESH PRODUCE

Asparagus	Cauliflower	Onions
Avocado	Celery	Radishes
Bell Peppers	Cucumber	Salad Mix
Berries	Eggplant	Squash
Broccoli	Fennel	Tomatoes
Brussel Sprouts	Garlic	Bok Choi
Cabbage	Green Beans	Chives
Carrots	Mushrooms	Spinach

MEAT AND SEAFOOD

Bacon	Lamb	Fish
Beef	Pork	Crab
Bison	Rotisserie Chicken	Lobster
Chicken	Sausage	Scallops
Deli meat	Turkey	Shrimp
Ground Beef / Ground Turkey	Oyster	Mussels

DAIRY PRODUCTS

Butter	Eggs	Sour Cream
Cheese	Greek Yogurt, full fat	Ghee
Cream Cheese	Heavy Whipping Cream	Mayo

PANTRY ITEMS

Avocado oil	Tea/Coffee	Moon Cheese
Beef Jerky	Pork Rinds	Low Carb Protein Bars
Bone Broth	Mayonnaise	All Natural Peanut Butter
Tuna, Salmon (canned)	Low Carb Salad Dressing	Stevia
Coconut Butter	Olive oil, extra virgin	Almonds
Coconut Oil	Olives	Spices
Almond Milk	Sweeteners	Almond Flour

FROZEN / OTHER

Low Carb Shopping List

FRESH PRODUCE

MEAT AND SEAFOOD

DAIRY PRODUCTS

PANTRY ITEMS

FROZEN / OTHER

Weekly Meal Planner

Week of: _____

	Breakfast	Lunch	Dinner	Snack	Notes
Monday	Carbs Fat Protein / TOTAL Cals	Carbs Fat Protein / TOTAL Cals	Carbs Fat Protein / TOTAL Cals	Carbs Fat Protein / TOTAL Cals	
Tuesday	Carbs Fat Protein / TOTAL Cals	Carbs Fat Protein / TOTAL Cals	Carbs Fat Protein / TOTAL Cals	Carbs Fat Protein / TOTAL Cals	
Wednesday	Carbs Fat Protein / TOTAL Cals	Carbs Fat Protein / TOTAL Cals	Carbs Fat Protein / TOTAL Cals	Carbs Fat Protein / TOTAL Cals	
Thursday	Carbs Fat Protein / TOTAL Cals	Carbs Fat Protein / TOTAL Cals	Carbs Fat Protein / TOTAL Cals	Carbs Fat Protein / TOTAL Cals	
Friday	Carbs Fat Protein / TOTAL Cals	Carbs Fat Protein / TOTAL Cals	Carbs Fat Protein / TOTAL Cals	Carbs Fat Protein / TOTAL Cals	
Saturday	Carbs Fat Protein / TOTAL Cals	Carbs Fat Protein / TOTAL Cals	Carbs Fat Protein / TOTAL Cals	Carbs Fat Protein / TOTAL Cals	
Sunday	Carbs Fat Protein / TOTAL Cals	Carbs Fat Protein / TOTAL Cals	Carbs Fat Protein / TOTAL Cals	Carbs Fat Protein / TOTAL Cals	

Keto Grocery Inventory

DATE: _____

QTY	PRODUCE

QTY	MEAT & FISH

QTY	FROZEN FOODS

QTY	DAIRY

QTY	PANTRY

QTY	OTHER/MISC.

Low Carb Grocery Ideas

FRESH PRODUCE

☐ Asparagus	☐ Cauliflower	☐ Onions
☐ Avocado	☐ Celery	☐ Radishes
☐ Bell Peppers	☐ Cucumber	☐ Salad Mix
☐ Berries	☐ Eggplant	☐ Squash
☐ Broccoli	☐ Fennel	☐ Tomatoes
☐ Brussel Sprouts	☐ Garlic	☐ Bok Choi
☐ Cabbage	☐ Green Beans	☐ Chives
☐ Carrots	☐ Mushrooms	☐ Spinach

MEAT AND SEAFOOD

☐ Bacon	☐ Lamb	☐ Fish
☐ Beef	☐ Pork	☐ Crab
☐ Bison	☐ Rotisserie Chicken	☐ Lobster
☐ Chicken	☐ Sausage	☐ Scallops
☐ Deli meat	☐ Turkey	☐ Shrimp
☐ Ground Beef / Ground Turkey	☐ Oyster	☐ Mussels

DAIRY PRODUCTS

☐ Butter	☐ Eggs	☐ Sour Cream
☐ Cheese	☐ Greek Yogurt, full fat	☐ Ghee
☐ Cream Cheese	☐ Heavy Whipping Cream	☐ Mayo

PANTRY ITEMS

☐ Avocado oil	☐ Tea/Coffee	☐ Moon Cheese
☐ Beef Jerky	☐ Pork Rinds	☐ Low Carb Protein Bars
☐ Bone Broth	☐ Mayonnaise	☐ All Natural Peanut Butter
☐ Tuna, Salmon (canned)	☐ Low Carb Salad Dressing	☐ Stevia
☐ Coconut Butter	☐ Olive oil, extra virgin	☐ Almonds
☐ Coconut Oil	☐ Olives	☐ Spices
☐ Almond Milk	☐ Sweeteners	☐ Almond Flour

FROZEN / OTHER

☐	☐	☐
☐	☐	☐
☐	☐	☐
☐	☐	☐

Low Carb Shopping List

FRESH PRODUCE

MEAT AND SEAFOOD

DAIRY PRODUCTS

PANTRY ITEMS

FROZEN / OTHER

Weekly Meal Planner

Week of: _____

	Breakfast	Lunch	Dinner	Snack	Notes
Monday	Carbs Fat Protein TOTAL Cals	Carbs Fat Protein TOTAL Cals	Carbs Fat Protein TOTAL Cals	Carbs Fat Protein TOTAL Cals	
Tuesday	Carbs Fat Protein TOTAL Cals	Carbs Fat Protein TOTAL Cals	Carbs Fat Protein TOTAL Cals	Carbs Fat Protein TOTAL Cals	
Wednesday	Carbs Fat Protein TOTAL Cals	Carbs Fat Protein TOTAL Cals	Carbs Fat Protein TOTAL Cals	Carbs Fat Protein TOTAL Cals	
Thursday	Carbs Fat Protein TOTAL Cals	Carbs Fat Protein TOTAL Cals	Carbs Fat Protein TOTAL Cals	Carbs Fat Protein TOTAL Cals	
Friday	Carbs Fat Protein TOTAL Cals	Carbs Fat Protein TOTAL Cals	Carbs Fat Protein TOTAL Cals	Carbs Fat Protein TOTAL Cals	
Saturday	Carbs Fat Protein TOTAL Cals	Carbs Fat Protein TOTAL Cals	Carbs Fat Protein TOTAL Cals	Carbs Fat Protein TOTAL Cals	
Sunday	Carbs Fat Protein TOTAL Cals	Carbs Fat Protein TOTAL Cals	Carbs Fat Protein TOTAL Cals	Carbs Fat Protein TOTAL Cals	

Keto Grocery Inventory

DATE: _____

QTY	PRODUCE

QTY	MEAT & FISH

QTY	FROZEN FOODS

QTY	DAIRY

QTY	PANTRY

QTY	OTHER/MISC.

Low Carb Grocery Ideas

FRESH PRODUCE

☐ Asparagus	☐ Cauliflower	☐ Onions
☐ Avocado	☐ Celery	☐ Radishes
☐ Bell Peppers	☐ Cucumber	☐ Salad Mix
☐ Berries	☐ Eggplant	☐ Squash
☐ Broccoli	☐ Fennel	☐ Tomatoes
☐ Brussel Sprouts	☐ Garlic	☐ Bok Choi
☐ Cabbage	☐ Green Beans	☐ Chives
☐ Carrots	☐ Mushrooms	☐ Spinach

MEAT AND SEAFOOD

☐ Bacon	☐ Lamb	☐ Fish
☐ Beef	☐ Pork	☐ Crab
☐ Bison	☐ Rotisserie Chicken	☐ Lobster
☐ Chicken	☐ Sausage	☐ Scallops
☐ Deli meat	☐ Turkey	☐ Shrimp
☐ Ground Beef / Ground Turkey	☐ Oyster	☐ Mussels

DAIRY PRODUCTS

☐ Butter	☐ Eggs	☐ Sour Cream
☐ Cheese	☐ Greek Yogurt, full fat	☐ Ghee
☐ Cream Cheese	☐ Heavy Whipping Cream	☐ Mayo

PANTRY ITEMS

☐ Avocado oil	☐ Tea/Coffee	☐ Moon Cheese
☐ Beef Jerky	☐ Pork Rinds	☐ Low Carb Protein Bars
☐ Bone Broth	☐ Mayonnaise	☐ All Natural Peanut Butter
☐ Tuna, Salmon (canned)	☐ Low Carb Salad Dressing	☐ Stevia
☐ Coconut Butter	☐ Olive oil, extra virgin	☐ Almonds
☐ Coconut Oil	☐ Olives	☐ Spices
☐ Almond Milk	☐ Sweeteners	☐ Almond Flour

FROZEN / OTHER

☐	☐	☐
☐	☐	☐
☐	☐	☐
☐	☐	☐

Low Carb Shopping List

FRESH PRODUCE

MEAT AND SEAFOOD

DAIRY PRODUCTS

PANTRY ITEMS

FROZEN / OTHER

Weekly Meal Planner

Week of: _____

	Breakfast	Lunch	Dinner	Snack	Notes
Monday	Carbs Fat Protein TOTAL Cals	Carbs Fat Protein TOTAL Cals	Carbs Fat Protein TOTAL Cals	Carbs Fat Protein TOTAL Cals	
Tuesday	Carbs Fat Protein TOTAL Cals	Carbs Fat Protein TOTAL Cals	Carbs Fat Protein TOTAL Cals	Carbs Fat Protein TOTAL Cals	
Wednesday	Carbs Fat Protein TOTAL Cals	Carbs Fat Protein TOTAL Cals	Carbs Fat Protein TOTAL Cals	Carbs Fat Protein TOTAL Cals	
Thursday	Carbs Fat Protein TOTAL Cals	Carbs Fat Protein TOTAL Cals	Carbs Fat Protein TOTAL Cals	Carbs Fat Protein TOTAL Cals	
Friday	Carbs Fat Protein TOTAL Cals	Carbs Fat Protein TOTAL Cals	Carbs Fat Protein TOTAL Cals	Carbs Fat Protein TOTAL Cals	
Saturday	Carbs Fat Protein TOTAL Cals	Carbs Fat Protein TOTAL Cals	Carbs Fat Protein TOTAL Cals	Carbs Fat Protein TOTAL Cals	
Sunday	Carbs Fat Protein TOTAL Cals	Carbs Fat Protein TOTAL Cals	Carbs Fat Protein TOTAL Cals	Carbs Fat Protein TOTAL Cals	

Keto Grocery Inventory

DATE: _____

QTY	PRODUCE

QTY	MEAT & FISH

QTY	FROZEN FOODS

QTY	DAIRY

QTY	PANTRY

QTY	OTHER/MISC.

Low Carb Grocery Ideas

FRESH PRODUCE

Asparagus		Cauliflower		Onions	
Avocado		Celery		Radishes	
Bell Peppers		Cucumber		Salad Mix	
Berries		Eggplant		Squash	
Broccoli		Fennel		Tomatoes	
Brussel Sprouts		Garlic		Bok Choi	
Cabbage		Green Beans		Chives	
Carrots		Mushrooms		Spinach	

MEAT AND SEAFOOD

Bacon	Lamb	Fish	
Beef	Pork	Crab	
Bison	Rotisserie Chicken	Lobster	
Chicken	Sausage	Scallops	
Deli meat	Turkey	Shrimp	
Ground Beef / Ground Turkey	Oyster	Mussels	

DAIRY PRODUCTS

Butter	Eggs	Sour Cream
Cheese	Greek Yogurt, full fat	Ghee
Cream Cheese	Heavy Whipping Cream	Mayo

PANTRY ITEMS

Avocado oil	Tea/Coffee	Moon Cheese
Beef Jerky	Pork Rinds	Low Carb Protein Bars
Bone Broth	Mayonnaise	All Natural Peanut Butter
Tuna, Salmon (canned)	Low Carb Salad Dressing	Stevia
Coconut Butter	Olive oil, extra virgin	Almonds
Coconut Oil	Olives	Spices
Almond Milk	Sweeteners	Almond Flour

FROZEN / OTHER

Low Carb Shopping List

FRESH PRODUCE

MEAT AND SEAFOOD

DAIRY PRODUCTS

PANTRY ITEMS

FROZEN / OTHER

Printed in Great Britain
by Amazon